2023 Ultimate Fat Loss Handbook:

A Straightforward, No-Nonsense Guide

Minnie D. Fanning

Table of Contents

<u>Summing up the key principles of this book</u>
<u>Empowering you to achieve your fat loss goals.</u>

1.Introduction

Once upon a time, there was a woman named Sarah who had struggled with her weight for as long as she could remember. She had tried every diet and exercise plan under the sun, but nothing seemed to stick. She felt discouraged and hopeless until one day, she stumbled upon a book titled "The Ultimate Fat Loss Handbook: A Straightforward, No-Nonsense Guide" by Minnie D. Fanning on Amazon bookstore.

Intrigued by the title, Sarah decided to give it a shot and purchased the book. As she began reading, she was pleasantly surprised by how the author cut through all the misinformation and fad diets and focused on the science of fat loss. The book provided practical and actionable advice that she could easily follow.

Sarah eagerly put the tips and tricks she learned into practice and was amazed by the results. She started to see her weight drop, her energy levels increase, and her confidence soar. She felt empowered and in control of her health for the first time in her life.

In no time, Sarah had reached her goal weight and was maintaining it with ease. She was grateful to have found "The Ultimate Fat Loss Handbook" and couldn't imagine ever going back to her old ways. She recommended the book to all of her friends and family, who also had success with its guidance.

From that day on, Sarah lived a happy and healthy life, thanks to the knowledge she gained from "The Ultimate Fat Loss Handbook."

The problem with traditional weight loss approaches

Traditional weight loss approaches often rely on strict diets, elimination of certain foods or food groups, and excessive exercise. These methods can be difficult to maintain in the long term and often result in yo-yo dieting, where individuals repeatedly lose weight only to gain it back.

Additionally, traditional approaches often focus on quick fixes and short-term solutions rather than addressing the underlying causes of weight gain. This can lead to a lack of understanding about the science of fat loss and how the body responds to changes in nutrition and exercise.

Another issue with traditional weight loss approaches is that they can be overly restrictive and unrealistic, leading to feelings of deprivation and a lack of enjoyment in eating. This can lead to binge eating, decreased motivation, and ultimately, failure.

Moreover, traditional weight loss approaches do not take into account individual differences such as genetics, body type, and metabolism, making a one-size-fits-all approach ineffective for many people.

Overall, traditional weight loss approaches often lead to frustration, disappointment, and a lack of lasting results. It's important to adopt a more holistic and sustainable approach to weight loss that focuses on a balanced and nutritious diet, regular exercise, and lifestyle changes that can be maintained for life.

The focus of this book

The focus of this book, "The Ultimate Fat Loss Handbook: A Straightforward, No-Nonsense Guide," is to provide a scientifically-based and practical approach to weight loss that is both achievable and sustainable.

The book cuts through the noise and misinformation of traditional weight loss approaches and focuses on the science of fat loss, providing a clear understanding of how the body loses weight and the role of nutrition and exercise in the process.

The book also emphasizes the importance of setting realistic goals, tracking progress, and incorporating healthy lifestyle changes that can be maintained for life.

Throughout the book, readers will learn about the power of nutrition, including the truth about calories and macronutrients, the role of the glycemic index and load, and how to incorporate healthy and whole foods into their diet.

In addition, the book provides practical tips and tricks for exercise, including the benefits of strength training and cardio, developing a balanced exercise plan, and incorporating high-intensity interval training.

This book also addresses common barriers to weight loss and provides strategies for overcoming cravings and emotional eating, dealing with plateaus, and staying motivated and accountable.

Ultimately, the focus of this book is to empower readers with the knowledge and tools they need to achieve their weight loss goals and maintain a healthy weight for life.

II. Understanding the Science of Fat Loss

Understanding the science of fat loss is critical for achieving long-term weight loss success. The process of fat loss involves multiple physiological and hormonal factors that work together to determine the amount of fat stored in the body and the rate at which it is burned for energy.

One key factor is calorie balance, which refers to the balance between the number of calories consumed through food and the number of calories burned through physical activity and basic metabolic processes. To lose weight, it is necessary to create a calorie deficit, meaning that you must consume fewer calories than you burn.

Another important factor is the role of nutrition, specifically the balance of macronutrients (carbohydrates, protein, and fat) in the diet. Different macronutrients have different effects on hormones and metabolism, and the right balance can support weight loss and improve overall health.

Exercise also plays a crucial role in the science of fat loss. Physical activity helps increase energy expenditure, promote muscle development, and support a healthy metabolism. In addition, strength training and high-intensity interval training have been shown to be particularly effective for fat loss.

It is also important to understand the role of hormones in fat loss. Hormones such as insulin, leptin, and cortisol can impact the body's ability to store and burn fat. A diet high in processed and sugary foods, for example, can lead to insulin resistance and decreased fat oxidation, making it more difficult to lose weight.

In conclusion, the science of fat loss involves multiple complex factors that interact with each other to determine the amount of fat stored in the body and the rate at which it is burned. By understanding the science and how to create a calorie deficit, maintain a balanced diet, and incorporate regular exercise, individuals can achieve their weight loss goals and maintain a healthy weight for life.

How the body loses weight

The body loses weight when it burns more calories than it consumes. This creates a calorie deficit, which leads to a reduction in the amount of stored energy in the form of fat.

The process of weight loss begins when the body starts to break down stored fat for energy. Fat cells, also known as adipocytes, contain stored triglycerides, which are composed of fatty acids and glycerol. When the body needs energy and glucose levels are low, the hormone insulin decreases, and the stored triglycerides are broken down into fatty acids and glycerol. These fatty acids are then transported to the muscle cells, where they are burned for energy.

Exercise and physical activity increase the rate at which the body burns calories and can help create a calorie deficit, leading to weight loss. Resistance training, in particular, can increase muscle mass, which can help boost the metabolism and promote weight loss.

In addition to exercise, nutrition also plays a crucial role in the body's ability to lose weight. A diet high in whole, nutrient-dense foods, such as vegetables, fruits, and lean protein, can help support weight loss and improve overall health. A diet high in processed and sugary foods, on the other hand, can lead to hormonal imbalances and decreased fat oxidation, making it more difficult to lose weight.

It's important to remember that weight loss is a slow and gradual process, and it's not uncommon to experience plateaus and setbacks along the way. However, by focusing on a balanced diet and regular exercise, and by being patient and persistent, individuals can achieve their weight loss goals and maintain a healthy weight for life.

The role of nutrition and exercise

Nutrition and exercise are both crucial components of a successful weight loss program. The body loses weight when it burns more calories than it consumes, and a balanced diet and regular exercise can help support this process.

Nutrition is essential for weight loss because it provides the body with the energy and nutrients it needs to function properly. A balanced diet that includes a variety of whole, nutrient-dense foods, such as vegetables, fruits, and lean protein, can help support weight loss and improve overall health. On the other hand, a diet high in processed and sugary foods can lead to hormonal imbalances and decreased fat oxidation, making it more difficult to lose weight.

Exercise is also important for weight loss because it helps increase energy expenditure and promotes muscle development. Regular physical activity, especially resistance training, can increase muscle mass, which can help boost the metabolism and promote weight loss. In addition, high-intensity interval training (HIIT) has been shown to be particularly effective for fat loss.

It's important to remember that weight loss is a slow and gradual process, and it's not uncommon to experience plateaus and setbacks along the way. By incorporating both a balanced diet and regular exercise into their routine, individuals can increase their chances of success and maintain a healthy weight for life.

In conclusion, the role of nutrition and exercise in weight loss is complex and intertwined. A balanced diet that provides the body with the energy and nutrients it needs, combined with regular physical activity, is essential for achieving and maintaining a healthy weight.

The importance of hormones and metabolism

Hormones and metabolism play a crucial role in weight loss and overall health. Hormones are chemical messengers produced by the endocrine glands, and they regulate many of the body's processes, including appetite, metabolism, and fat storage.

The metabolism is the process by which the body converts food into energy. The rate at which the body burns calories, known as the metabolic rate, is influenced by several factors, including hormones, genetics, and physical activity.

Hormones such as insulin, leptin, and cortisol play a key role in regulating metabolism and fat storage. Insulin is a hormone produced by the pancreas that regulates glucose levels in the blood. When insulin levels are high, the body is more likely to store fat, and when insulin levels are low, the body is more likely to burn stored fat for energy.

Leptin is a hormone produced by fat cells that regulates energy balance and hunger. When leptin levels are high, the body is more likely to burn stored fat, and when leptin levels are low, the body is more likely to store fat.

Cortisol is a stress hormone produced by the adrenal glands. Chronic stress can lead to elevated cortisol levels, which can lead to increased fat storage and decreased fat burning.

In addition to hormones, genetics also play a role in metabolism and weight loss. Some individuals may have a slower metabolism, making it more challenging for them to lose weight, while others may have a faster metabolism, making it easier for them to lose weight.

It's important to understand the role of hormones and metabolism in weight loss because this knowledge can help individuals make informed decisions about their diet and exercise routines. By making lifestyle changes that support hormonal balance and healthy metabolism, individuals can increase their chances of success in achieving and maintaining a healthy weight.

III. Setting Realistic Goals

Setting realistic goals is an important step in the weight loss journey. Unrealistic expectations can lead to frustration, disappointment, and eventually give up. On the other hand, achievable goals can provide motivation, build confidence, and increase the likelihood of success.

When setting weight loss goals, it's important to be specific and measurable. For example, instead of setting a goal to "lose weight," set a goal to "lose 10 pounds in the next 12 weeks." Having a specific target in mind makes it easier to track progress and stay motivated.

It's also important to set achievable goals that are based on a healthy rate of weight loss. A safe and healthy rate of weight loss is generally considered to be 1-2 pounds per week. Losing weight too quickly can be unhealthy and may not be sustainable in the long term.

In addition to setting specific and achievable goals, it's important to be realistic about the time and effort required to achieve those goals. Losing weight and maintaining a healthy weight takes time and effort, and it's important to have a plan in place for both diet and exercise.

Finally, it's important to set both short-term and long-term goals. Short-term goals can provide immediate motivation, while long-term goals can help keep individuals on track and focused on the end goal.

In conclusion, setting realistic goals is essential for success in the weight loss journey. By being specific, measurable, achievable, and realistic, individuals can increase their chances of success and stay motivated on the path to a healthier weight.

Understanding your body type and starting point

Understanding your body type and starting point is an important step in the weight loss journey. Every individual is unique, and factors such as genetics, body composition, and past lifestyle habits play a role in determining starting weight and body type.

There are three main body types: ectomorph, mesomorph, and endomorph. Ectomorphs are naturally thin and have a fast metabolism, making it easier for them to lose weight. Mesomorphs have a balanced metabolism and can gain and lose weight relatively easily. Endomorphs have a slow metabolism and tend to store fat easily, making it more challenging for them to lose weight.

It's important to understand your body type because this knowledge can help you tailor your diet and exercise routine to meet your specific needs. For example, endomorphs may need to focus on reducing calorie intake and increasing physical activity to see results, while ectomorphs may need to focus on building muscle mass through strength training.

In addition to understanding body type, it's important to have a clear understanding of your starting point. This includes your current weight, body fat percentage, and any health conditions that may affect your weight loss journey.

By understanding your body type and starting point, individuals can make informed decisions about their diet and exercise routines and increase their chances of success in achieving and maintaining a healthy weight.

Setting achievable and sustainable goals

Setting achievable and sustainable goals is a critical step in the weight loss journey. Goals that are too unrealistic or unsustainable can lead to frustration, disappointment, and eventually, giving up. On the other hand, achievable and sustainable goals can provide motivation, build confidence, and increase the likelihood of success.

When setting weight loss goals, it's important to be specific and measurable. For example, instead of setting a goal to "lose weight," set a goal to "lose 10 pounds in the next 12 weeks." Having a specific target in mind makes it easier to track progress and stay motivated.

It's also important to set achievable goals that are based on a healthy rate of weight loss. A safe and healthy rate of weight loss is generally considered to be 1-2 pounds per week. Losing weight too quickly can be unhealthy and may not be sustainable in the long term.

In addition to being achievable, goals must also be sustainable. This means making lifestyle changes that can be maintained in the long term. Rapid weight loss through crash diets or extreme exercise routines is not sustainable and is likely to result in weight regain. Instead, individuals should focus on making gradual, achievable changes to their diet and exercise routines that can be maintained in the long term.

Finally, it's important to have a plan in place for achieving and maintaining your goals. This includes making changes to your diet, increasing physical activity, and seeking support from friends, family, or a healthcare professional.

In conclusion, setting achievable and sustainable goals is essential for success in the weight loss journey. By being specific, measurable, achievable, and sustainable, individuals can increase their chances of success and stay motivated on the path to a healthier weight.

Tracking your progress

Tracking your progress is an important step in the weight loss journey. It allows individuals to see the results of their efforts and make adjustments to their diet and exercise routines as needed. Regular monitoring also provides motivation and a sense of accomplishment, as individuals can see the progress they are making towards their goals.

There are several ways to track progress, including:

Weighing yourself: Weighing yourself regularly, perhaps once a week, is a simple and effective way to track progress. It's important to weigh yourself at the same time each day, preferably first thing in the morning after using the bathroom, and to use the same scale.

Measuring body fat percentage: In addition to weighing yourself, measuring body fat percentage can provide a more comprehensive picture of progress. Body fat percentage measures the amount of fat in your body, as opposed to weight, which includes muscle, bone, and other tissues. Body fat percentage can be measured using skin fold calipers, bioelectrical impedance, or dual-energy x-ray absorptiometry (DXA) scans.

Taking progress photos: Taking progress photos is a visual way to track progress. By comparing photos taken at different points in time, individuals can see the changes in their body shape and size.

Keeping a food diary: Keeping a food diary can help individuals track their calorie intake and monitor their progress. This can also help individuals identify any areas where they need to make changes, such as reducing portion sizes or choosing healthier food options.

Monitoring physical activity: Tracking physical activity, such as the number of steps taken or minutes of exercise completed each day, can provide insight into progress and help individuals stay on track.

In conclusion, tracking progress is an important step in the weight loss journey. By regularly monitoring weight, body fat percentage, physical activity, and food intake, individuals can see the results of their efforts and make informed decisions about their diet and exercise routines.

IV. The Power of Nutrition

Nutrition plays a crucial role in the weight loss journey. What we eat affects our energy levels, our metabolism, and our overall health. By making informed food choices, individuals can increase their chances of success and achieve their weight loss goals.

Eating a balanced diet that includes a variety of nutrient-dense foods, such as fruits, vegetables, whole grains, and lean proteins, can help individuals feel full and satisfied while still managing their calorie intake. It's also important to limit the intake of processed and high-calorie foods, such as junk food and sugary drinks, which can contribute to weight gain.

In addition to eating a balanced diet, individuals can also make strategic food choices to support their weight loss goals. For example, consuming foods that are high in fiber, such as fruits, vegetables, and whole grains, can help individuals feel full and reduce overall calorie intake. Eating protein-rich foods, such as lean meats, poultry, fish, and beans, can also help individuals feel full and preserve muscle mass, which is essential for weight loss.

It's also important to be mindful of portion sizes. Consuming large portions, even of healthy foods, can still lead to weight gain if calorie intake exceeds the amount of energy burned.

In conclusion, nutrition plays a crucial role in the weight loss journey. By making informed food choices, eating a balanced diet, and being mindful of portion sizes, individuals can support their weight loss goals and achieve success.

The truth about calories and macronutrients

Calories and macronutrients are important factors to consider when it comes to weight loss. Understanding how these elements affect the body can help individuals make informed choices and achieve their goals.

Calories are units of energy that are used to fuel the body. The number of calories an individual needs each day depends on several factors, including age, gender, weight, height, and activity level. To lose weight, individuals need to create a calorie deficit, which means they need to burn more calories than they consume.

Macronutrients, on the other hand, are the three key components of food: carbohydrates, proteins, and fats. Each of these macronutrients plays a unique role in the body and can impact weight loss differently.

Carbohydrates are the body's primary source of energy and are found in foods such as bread, pasta, rice, fruits, and vegetables. While carbohydrates are important for fueling the body, consuming too many can lead to weight gain.

Proteins are essential for building and repairing tissues in the body, as well as maintaining muscle mass. Foods that are high in protein include meat, poultry, fish, beans, and dairy products.

Fats, while often demonized, are an essential component of a healthy diet. Fats help the body absorb certain vitamins and minerals, as well as provide energy. However, it's important to choose healthy fats, such as those found in nuts, seeds, avocados, and olive oil, and limit the intake of unhealthy fats, such as those found in fried foods and processed snacks.

In conclusion, calories and macronutrients play an important role in weight loss. Understanding how these elements affect the body, as well as making informed food choices, can help individuals achieve their goals and maintain a healthy weight.

Understanding the glycemic index and load

The glycemic index (GI) and glycemic load (GL) are important concepts to understand when it comes to weight loss and healthy eating. These terms refer to the impact that carbohydrates have on blood sugar levels.

The glycemic index is a rating system that measures how quickly carbohydrates raise blood sugar levels after they are consumed. Foods are rated on a scale of 0 to 100, with higher numbers indicating a quicker rise in blood sugar levels. Foods with a high GI are rapidly absorbed and cause a rapid spike in blood sugar levels, while foods with a low GI are absorbed more slowly and have a more gradual impact on blood sugar levels.

The glycemic load, on the other hand, measures the total impact of a food on blood sugar levels. It takes into account both the GI and the amount of carbohydrates in a serving of food. Foods with a high GL can cause a rapid and significant rise in blood sugar levels, while foods with a low GL have a more gradual and modest impact.

Why is this important for weight loss? Foods that cause rapid spikes in blood sugar levels can also lead to rapid spikes in insulin, which is the hormone responsible for regulating blood sugar levels. When insulin levels are elevated, the body is less likely to burn fat for energy and more likely to store fat. This can lead to weight gain and make it more difficult to lose weight.

In conclusion, understanding the glycemic index and glycemic load can be a helpful tool in managing weight and supporting weight loss goals. By choosing foods that have a low GI and GL, individuals can help regulate their blood sugar levels, control insulin levels, and promote fat burning.

Incorporating healthy and whole foods into your diet

Incorporating healthy and whole foods into your diet is a key component of achieving and maintaining a healthy weight. Whole foods are unprocessed or minimally processed foods that are closest to their natural state and provide a wealth of nutrients, vitamins, and minerals.

Healthy and whole foods, such as fruits, vegetables, whole grains, lean proteins, and healthy fats, are not only more nutritious but are also often lower in calories, making them ideal for weight loss. By replacing processed and high-calorie foods with healthier options, individuals can reduce their calorie intake and promote weight loss.

Incorporating more fruits and vegetables into the diet is a simple way to boost nutrition and support weight loss goals. Fruits and vegetables are low in calories and high in fiber, which can help individuals feel full and reduce overall calorie intake. Additionally, many fruits and vegetables are high in water content, which can also contribute to feelings of fullness.

Whole grains, such as brown rice, whole wheat bread, and quinoa, are also an important part of a healthy diet. Unlike refined grains, which are stripped of their nutrients, whole grains provide a rich source of fiber, vitamins, and minerals.

Incorporating lean proteins, such as chicken, fish, and legumes, can also help support weight loss goals. Proteins are more filling than carbohydrates and can help regulate hunger and control cravings.

Finally, incorporating healthy fats, such as those found in nuts, seeds, avocados, and olive oil, can help support weight loss by providing energy and helping to regulate hormones.

In conclusion, incorporating healthy and whole foods into your diet can play a critical role in achieving and maintaining a healthy weight. By replacing processed and high-calorie foods with healthier options, individuals can support their weight loss goals, improve their overall nutrition, and achieve a healthier, more sustainable diet.

The role of supplementation and hydration

Supplementation and hydration are important components of a healthy weight loss program. While a healthy diet and exercise program are the foundation of weight loss, supplementation and hydration can support these efforts and help individuals achieve their goals more effectively.

Supplementation can be an effective tool for weight loss when used in conjunction with a healthy diet and exercise program. Some supplements, such as protein powders, fiber supplements, and fat-burning supplements, can help support weight loss by providing additional nutrition, reducing cravings, and increasing energy levels.

However, it's important to keep in mind that supplements should never be used as a replacement for a healthy diet and exercise program. Instead, they should be used to supplement these efforts and support weight loss goals. Additionally, it's important to consult with a healthcare professional before starting any new supplement regimen, as some supplements may interact with medications or have other potential side effects.

Hydration is also critical to weight loss. Proper hydration is important for maintaining health, regulating metabolism, and supporting weight loss efforts. Drinking plenty of water throughout the day can help individuals feel full and reduce cravings, while also flushing out toxins and supporting overall health.

In conclusion, supplementation and hydration can play a supportive role in weight loss efforts. When used in conjunction with a healthy diet and exercise program, they can help individuals achieve their weight loss goals and support their overall health and well-being. However, it's important to use these tools wisely and consult with a healthcare professional when necessary.

V. Exercise for Effective Fat Loss

Exercise is an essential component of effective fat loss. Regular physical activity not only helps to burn calories, but also promotes muscle growth, improves metabolism, and supports overall health and well-being.

For fat loss, it is important to engage in both cardiovascular exercise and resistance training. Cardiovascular exercise, such as running, cycling, or swimming, is important for burning calories and promoting fat loss. Resistance training, such as weightlifting, bodyweight exercises, or resistance bands, is important for building muscle, which in turn can boost metabolism and support weight loss.

Incorporating both types of exercise into your routine can be an effective way to support fat loss efforts. For example, a workout routine that includes 30 minutes of cardio followed by 30 minutes of resistance training can be an effective way to burn calories and promote weight loss.

It is also important to make exercise a sustainable part of your routine. Regular physical activity, at least three to four times a week, is crucial for maintaining health and supporting weight loss efforts.

Finally, it's important to challenge yourself and gradually increase intensity and duration to prevent plateaus and promote continued progress. This can be achieved by gradually increasing the weight used during resistance training, or by incorporating intervals or high-intensity training into your cardio routine.

In conclusion, exercise is an important component of effective fat loss. Incorporating both cardiovascular and resistance training into your routine, making exercise a sustainable part of your routine, and gradually increasing intensity and duration can help support fat loss efforts and promote overall health and well-being.

The benefits of strength training and cardio

Strength training and cardio are both important forms of exercise that offer unique benefits for weight loss and overall health.

Strength training, which includes exercises such as weightlifting, bodyweight exercises, and resistance bands, can help build muscle and boost metabolism. This increased muscle mass burns more calories, even when at rest, helping to support weight loss efforts. In addition, strength training can help improve posture, increase bone density, and reduce the risk of injury.

Cardiovascular exercise, such as running, cycling, swimming, or any other activity that raises the heart rate for an extended period, is crucial for burning calories and promoting fat loss. Cardio can help improve cardiovascular health, increase endurance, and reduce the risk of chronic disease.

While both strength training and cardio have unique benefits, incorporating both into your exercise routine can provide even greater benefits. Strength training can help build muscle and boost metabolism, while cardio can help burn calories and improve cardiovascular health. When combined, these two forms of exercise can help create a well-rounded fitness program that supports weight loss and overall health.

In conclusion, strength training and cardio both offer unique benefits for weight loss and overall health. Incorporating both into your exercise routine can provide even greater benefits and help create a well-rounded fitness program. Whether you prefer strength training, cardio, or a combination of both, it is important to make regular physical activity a sustainable part of your routine.

Developing a balanced exercise plan

Developing a balanced exercise plan is crucial for achieving weight loss and maintaining overall health. A balanced exercise plan should include a combination of strength training and cardio, as well as stretching and recovery activities.

Strength training, such as weightlifting, bodyweight exercises, or resistance bands, should be performed two to three times a week, focusing on different muscle groups each time. Cardiovascular exercise, such as running, cycling, or swimming, should be performed at least three times a week, with the frequency and duration gradually increasing over time.

It's also important to incorporate stretching and recovery activities into your exercise plan. Stretching can help improve flexibility, reduce the risk of injury, and improve muscle imbalances. Recovery activities, such as yoga or foam rolling, can help reduce muscle soreness and promote overall recovery.

In addition to balancing different forms of exercise, it's important to also balance intensity and duration. Overdoing it on intense exercise can lead to injury, burnout, and decreased progress. On the other hand, not pushing yourself enough can result in a plateau and decreased progress. Finding the right balance is key to achieving weight loss and overall health.

Finally, it's important to listen to your body and adjust your exercise plan as needed. It's normal for your body to need more or less recovery time as you progress, so it's important to be flexible and adjust your plan as needed.

In conclusion, developing a balanced exercise plan that includes a combination of strength training, cardio, stretching, and recovery activities is crucial for achieving weight loss and maintaining overall health. It's important to listen to your body and adjust your plan as needed to ensure you are pushing yourself enough to make progress, while also avoiding injury and burnout.

Incorporating high-intensity interval training

High-Intensity Interval Training (HIIT) is a popular form of exercise that can be effective for weight loss and overall health. HIIT involves alternating periods of intense activity with periods of rest, typically lasting anywhere from 15-30 minutes.

The high-intensity portions of HIIT can be performed through various exercises, such as running, cycling, jumping jacks, or burpees. These intense intervals help to boost metabolism, increase calorie burn, and improve cardiovascular health. The rest intervals provide a chance for recovery, allowing you to push yourself harder during the next intense interval.

One of the benefits of HIIT is its time-efficiency. HIIT workouts can be completed in less time compared to traditional steady-state cardio, making it a popular choice for those who are short on time. HIIT workouts can also be tailored to your fitness level, making it a versatile option for beginners and advanced fitness enthusiasts alike.

It's important to incorporate HIIT into a balanced exercise plan, as it should not be the only form of exercise. HIIT can be performed two to three times a week, with other forms of exercise, such as strength training and steady-state cardio, also being included in your exercise plan. Additionally, HIIT can be intense, so it's important to start slowly and gradually increase the intensity and duration over time.

In conclusion, HIIT is a popular and effective form of exercise for weight loss and overall health. Incorporating HIIT into a balanced exercise plan can help boost metabolism, increase calorie burn, and improve cardiovascular health. It's important to start slowly and gradually increase the intensity and duration over time, while also incorporating other forms of exercise into your routine.

VI. Overcoming Barriers and Staying Motivated

Overcoming barriers and staying motivated are important aspects of successful weight loss. Unfortunately, they can also be some of the biggest challenges to overcome. Here are some tips to help you overcome barriers and stay motivated:

Set achievable and realistic goals: Setting goals that are too ambitious can lead to frustration and disappointment, so it's important to set achievable and realistic goals. This will help you make steady progress and stay motivated along the way.

Track your progress: Keeping track of your progress can help you stay motivated, as you can see the progress you are making over time. This can be done through keeping a food diary, tracking your weight, or measuring your body measurements.

Surround yourself with support: Having a supportive network of family and friends can be extremely helpful in keeping you motivated and overcoming barriers. Consider joining a support group or working with a coach or therapist to help keep you accountable and motivated.

Celebrate your successes: Celebrating your successes, no matter how small, can help you stay motivated and stay focused on your goals. Recognize your progress and reward yourself for reaching milestones, such as trying a new healthy recipe or buying new workout gear.

Be flexible and adaptable: Life can throw unexpected obstacles in your way, so it's important to be flexible and adaptable. If you have a setback, try to focus on what you can do to overcome it, rather than dwelling on what went wrong.

Find what works for you: There is no one-size-fits-all approach to weight loss, so it's important to find what works for you. Experiment with different approaches to nutrition and exercise, and don't be afraid to make changes if what you're doing isn't working.

In conclusion, overcoming barriers and staying motivated are key components of successful weight loss. By setting achievable and realistic goals, tracking your progress, surrounding yourself with support, celebrating your successes, being flexible and adaptable, and finding what works for you, you can overcome barriers and stay motivated on your weight loss journey.

Dealing with cravings and emotional eating

Dealing with cravings and emotional eating is a common challenge for many people trying to lose weight. Here are some tips to help you overcome these challenges:

Identify triggers: Understanding what triggers your cravings and emotional eating can help you better manage them. Keep a journal to track when you experience cravings or emotional eating, and what was happening at the time.

Plan ahead: Having healthy snacks readily available can help you avoid reaching for unhealthy options when cravings strike. Planning ahead for meals and snacks can also help you stay on track and avoid reaching for junk food when you're in a hurry.

Practice mindfulness: Mindfulness can help you become more aware of your thoughts and emotions, and can help you better manage cravings and emotional eating. Try to focus on the present moment, and pay attention to physical sensations, such as hunger and fullness.

Find healthy alternatives: Finding healthy alternatives for your favorite junk foods can help you satisfy cravings in a healthier way. Try to find healthier versions of your favorite snacks, or try new healthy snacks to keep things interesting.

Address underlying emotional issues: Sometimes cravings and emotional eating are rooted in underlying emotional issues, such as stress, anxiety, or depression. Consider working with a therapist to help address these issues and develop healthier coping mechanisms.

Get enough sleep: Lack of sleep can trigger cravings and emotional eating, so it's important to get enough sleep each night. Aim for 7-9 hours of quality sleep each night to help you better manage cravings and emotional eating.

Stay active: Regular physical activity can help reduce stress and improve your mood, which can help reduce cravings and emotional eating. Find an activity you enjoy, such as hiking, yoga, or dance, and make it a regular part of your routine.

In conclusion, dealing with cravings and emotional eating is a common challenge for many people trying to lose weight. By identifying triggers, planning ahead, practicing mindfulness, finding healthy alternatives, addressing underlying emotional issues, getting enough sleep, and staying active, you can better manage cravings and emotional eating on your weight loss journey.

Overcoming plateaus and setbacks

Overcoming plateaus and setbacks is a common challenge for many people trying to lose weight. Here are some tips to help you overcome these challenges:

Re-evaluate your goals: Make sure your goals are realistic and achievable. If you're not seeing the results you want, it may be time to adjust your goals or your approach.

Track your progress: Keeping track of your progress can help you see where you are and where you need to go. Use a journal or a tracking app to log your food intake, physical activity, and weight.

Mix things up: Doing the same thing over and over again can lead to boredom and a plateau in your weight loss progress. Mix things up by trying new exercises, trying new recipes, or changing up your routine.

Get support: Having a support system can help you stay motivated and on track. Join a support group, work with a coach or personal trainer, or reach out to friends and family for support.

Don't give up: Setbacks and plateaus are a normal part of the weight loss journey. Don't give up if you don't see immediate results. Keep pushing forward and stay committed to your goals.

Celebrate your successes: Celebrating your successes, no matter how small, can help keep you motivated and on track. Give yourself a reward when you hit a milestone, such as a new outfit or a treat.

Take care of yourself: Taking care of yourself both physically and mentally is essential for overcoming setbacks and plateaus. Get enough sleep, eat a balanced diet, and make time for self-care.

In conclusion, overcoming plateaus and setbacks is a common challenge for many people trying to lose weight. By re-evaluating your goals, tracking your progress, mixing things up, getting support, not giving up, celebrating your successes, and taking care of yourself, you can overcome these challenges and continue on your weight loss journey.

Staying motivated and accountable

Staying motivated and accountable is key to achieving your weight loss goals. Here are some tips to help you stay motivated and accountable:

Set realistic goals: Make sure your goals are achievable and realistic. Setting unrealistic goals can lead to frustration and a lack of motivation.

Create a plan: Having a plan in place can help you stay focused and on track. Write down your goals, what you need to do to achieve them, and when you want to achieve them by.

Track your progress: Keeping track of your progress can help you stay motivated and accountable. Use a journal or a tracking app to log your food intake, physical activity, and weight.

Get support: Having a support system can help you stay motivated and accountable. Join a support group, work with a coach or personal trainer, or reach out to friends and family for support.

Celebrate your successes: Celebrating your successes, no matter how small, can help keep you motivated and accountable. Give yourself a reward when you hit a milestone, such as a new outfit or a treat.

Surround yourself with positive influences: Surrounding yourself with positive influences can help you stay motivated and accountable. Avoid negative people who bring you down and focus on spending time with people who support and encourage you.

Stay accountable: Hold yourself accountable for your actions and decisions. Take responsibility for your progress and setbacks, and don't make excuses.

In conclusion, staying motivated and accountable is key to achieving your weight loss goals. By setting realistic goals, creating a plan, tracking your progress, getting support, celebrating your successes, surrounding yourself with positive influences, and staying accountable, you can stay motivated and on track as you work towards your weight loss goals.

VII. Maintenance and Lifestyle Changes

Maintenance and lifestyle changes are critical components of long-term weight loss success. Here's what you need to know:

Maintenance is a lifelong commitment: Weight loss is not a one-time event, it's a lifelong commitment. You need to maintain your healthy habits to keep the weight off.

Gradual weight gain is normal: Gradual weight gain is normal and to be expected. Your body weight will fluctuate, and that's okay as long as it stays within a healthy range.

Keep tracking: Continuously track your progress and adjust your habits as needed to maintain your weight loss.

Continue to eat a balanced diet: Maintaining a balanced diet is crucial to maintaining weight loss. Make sure to eat a variety of nutritious foods and limit your intake of processed and high-calorie foods.

Keep exercising: Regular exercise is important for maintaining weight loss. Find an exercise routine that you enjoy and stick with it.

Focus on lifestyle changes, not quick fixes: Fad diets and quick fixes may provide temporary results, but they're not sustainable. Focus on making lifestyle changes that you can maintain in the long term.

Find balance: Find a balance between work, exercise, and leisure time. Make sure to set aside time for yourself and engage in activities that bring you joy.

Be kind to yourself: Don't beat yourself up if you slip up. Instead, focus on getting back on track and continue to make progress.

In conclusion, maintenance and lifestyle changes are critical components of long-term weight loss success. By continuously tracking your progress, eating a balanced diet, exercising regularly, focusing on lifestyle changes, finding balance, and being kind to yourself, you can maintain your weight loss and live a healthy and fulfilling life.

The importance of sustainability

The importance of sustainability in weight loss cannot be overstated. Losing weight is not just about achieving a certain number on the scale, it's about creating healthy habits that you can maintain for the rest of your life. Here's why sustainability is so important:

Long-term success: Sustainable weight loss focuses on making gradual, lasting changes to your diet and lifestyle that you can maintain for the rest of your life. This leads to long-term success, rather than short-term gains that are often followed by weight regain.

Better health: Sustainable weight loss approaches promote healthy habits that improve overall health, rather than just reducing body weight.

Improved self-esteem: Sustainable weight loss allows you to make positive changes to your life that you can be proud of and that contribute to a positive self-image.

Avoiding yo-yo dieting: Yo-yo dieting, or losing and regaining weight multiple times, can be harmful to your health and self-esteem. Sustainability helps you avoid this cycle and achieve lasting weight loss success.

Better quality of life: Sustainability helps you create healthy habits that improve your quality of life and contribute to overall happiness and well-being.

In conclusion, sustainability is a critical factor in weight loss success. By focusing on making gradual, lasting changes to your diet and lifestyle, you can achieve long-term success, better health, improved self-esteem, avoid yo-yo dieting, and improve your overall quality of life.

Making lasting lifestyle changes

Making lasting lifestyle changes is the key to sustainable weight loss. Here's how you can do it:

Start slow: Making too many changes too quickly can be overwhelming. Start by making small, manageable changes to your diet and exercise routine, and gradually build upon them as you become more comfortable.

Focus on habits: Rather than focusing on specific foods or diets, focus on creating healthy habits. This includes eating a balanced diet, drinking plenty of water, getting enough sleep, and engaging in regular physical activity.

Find what works for you: Everyone is different, so what works for one person may not work for another. Experiment to find the approach that works best for you and stick with it.

Surround yourself with support: Having a supportive network of friends and family members can help you stay on track and motivated. Consider joining a weight loss support group or finding an accountability partner.

Be consistent: Consistency is key when it comes to lifestyle changes. Make an effort to stick to your new habits every day, even when faced with challenges.

Celebrate your successes: Celebrate your progress, no matter how small. Recognizing your successes will help keep you motivated and on track.

In conclusion, making lasting lifestyle changes requires effort and dedication, but it's well worth it in the end. By starting slow, focusing on habits, finding what works for you, surrounding yourself with support, being consistent, and celebrating your successes, you can achieve sustainable weight loss and improve your overall quality of life.

Continuing to track progress and make adjustments

Continuing to track your progress and make adjustments is essential for maintaining your weight loss success. Here's what you should keep in mind:

Track your progress: Regularly measuring your weight, body fat percentage, and other relevant metrics can help you see how far you've come and make any necessary adjustments.

Be flexible: Don't be afraid to make changes to your diet and exercise routine if they're not working for you. Be open to trying new approaches and finding what works best for your body.

Listen to your body: Pay attention to how you feel and make adjustments as needed. If you're feeling fatigued or run down, consider reducing the intensity of your workouts or adjusting your diet.

Keep your goals in mind: Remember why you started your weight loss journey and keep your goals in mind. This will help you stay focused and motivated.

Stay positive: A positive attitude is key to success. Surround yourself with positive influences and focus on your successes, rather than your setbacks.

Celebrate milestones: Celebrating milestones, such as reaching a specific weight loss goal or completing a challenging workout, can help you stay motivated and inspired.

By tracking your progress, being flexible, listening to your body, keeping your goals in mind, staying positive, and celebrating milestones, you can continue to make adjustments and maintain your weight loss success. Remember, this is a journey, and it's important to be patient and persistent. With time and effort, you can achieve your weight loss goals and improve your overall health and well-being.

VII. Conclusion

In conclusion," The Ultimate Fat Loss Handbook: A Straightforward, No-Nonsense Guide" has provided a comprehensive and evidence-based approach to weight loss. By focusing on the science of fat loss, the role of nutrition and exercise, setting realistic and achievable goals, tracking progress, and making sustainable lifestyle changes, you have the tools to succeed.

Losing weight can be a challenging journey, but it doesn't have to be. By following the principles outlined in this book, you can overcome barriers, stay motivated, and make lasting changes to your health and well-being.

Remember, weight loss is not a one-size-fits-all approach, and what works for one person may not work for another. It's important to find what works best for you and be patient and persistent. With time and effort, you can achieve your weight loss goals and improve your overall health and well-being.

So, take what you've learned in this book and start your journey towards a healthier and happier you. Best of luck!

Summing up the key principles of this book

In this book, ".The Ultimate Fat Loss Handbook: A Straightforward, No-Nonsense Guide," several key principles were discussed to help you achieve your weight loss goals. These principles include:

Understanding the Science of Fat Loss: A deep dive into how the body loses weight and the role hormones and metabolism play in the process.

Setting Realistic Goals: An emphasis on understanding your body type and starting point, and setting achievable and sustainable goals.

The Power of Nutrition: An explanation of the truth about calories and macronutrients, the glycemic index and load, and the importance of incorporating healthy and whole foods into your diet.

Exercise for Effective Fat Loss: A discussion of the benefits of strength training and cardio, the importance of a balanced exercise plan, and incorporating high-intensity interval training.

Overcoming Barriers and Staying Motivated: Strategies for dealing with cravings and emotional eating, overcoming plateaus and setbacks, and staying motivated and accountable.

Maintenance and Lifestyle Changes: An emphasis on the importance of sustainability, making lasting lifestyle changes, and continuing to track progress and make adjustments.

By following these principles, you can develop a comprehensive and effective approach to weight loss. It is important to find what works best for you and be patient and persistent. With time and effort, you can achieve your weight loss goals and improve your overall health and well-being.

Empowering you to achieve your fat loss goals.

This book was written with the goal of empowering you to achieve your fat loss goals. By providing you with the latest information and practical tips, you will be able to make informed decisions and develop an effective plan to reach your desired weight.

We understand that losing weight can be challenging, but with the right guidance and support, it can also be a transformative and rewarding experience. Our aim is to provide you with the knowledge and tools you need to overcome the barriers and stay motivated on your weight loss journey.

You are in control of your own journey, and we believe that you have the power to make a positive change. Whether you're looking to lose a few pounds or make a significant transformation, this book will provide you with the information and strategies you need to achieve your goals.

We believe in empowering you to make the best choices for your body, and we are confident that you will find the information and insights in this book to be valuable and helpful. So let's get started on your journey to a healthier, happier you!